EAT SMART FOR LIFE

A GUIDE TO DEVELOPING HEALTHY EATING
BEHAVIORS

FUNCTIONAL HEALTH SERIES

SAM FURY

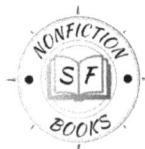

WARNINGS AND DISCLAIMERS

The information in this publication is made public for reference only.

Neither the author, publisher, nor anyone else involved in the production of this publication is responsible for how the reader uses the information or the result of his/her actions.

Nothing presented is medical advice. Implement anything you learn at your own risk. If in doubt, please consult a medical professional.

CONTENTS

This and all other books in the Functional Health Series, including the audiobook versions, are available at no extra cost inside our members area.

Get 30-days access for just $1!

www.functionalhealth.coach/members

INTRODUCTION

"Eat Smart for Life" offers essential knowledge and practical strategies for developing and maintaining healthy eating behaviors, a journey that can be both exciting and challenging. It begins by establishing an understanding of the fundamentals of nutrition, laying a foundation for making informed choices. Additionally, it offers insights into the drawbacks of fad diets, steering you toward healthier alternatives.

This naturally leads to a discussion on effective grocery shopping, where you'll find practical tips on how to choose ingredients that are beneficial for your health. These tips aim to make your trips to the grocery store less overwhelming and more productive.

Complementing the art of shopping, the guide also delves into meal planning and preparation. You will learn how to organize and prepare meals that are nutritious, enjoyable, and satisfying. These skills are crucial in creating a balanced diet that fits seamlessly into your lifestyle.

Addressing emotional eating and food cravings is another vital aspect of developing healthy eating habits. Understanding the triggers and learning strategies to manage these impulses is essential. In these sections, you will discover practical steps to overcome these challenges, helping you maintain your nutrition goals even in the face of temptation.

Dining out is a part of life, and this guide doesn't shy away from it. You'll learn how to make healthy choices in restaurants and social settings, enabling you to enjoy these experiences without compromising your nutrition goals. This extends to those on special diets, whether due to health conditions, allergies, or personal choices.

Each section of the guide is interconnected, building upon the previous to provide a comprehensive approach to healthy eating. The journey to a healthier you starts with understanding what you eat and why, and this guide is here to assist you every step of the way.

FUNDAMENTALS OF NUTRITION

First, let's explore the essential elements of a healthy diet. From macronutrients like proteins, carbohydrates, and fats to micronutrients like vitamins and minerals, we'll uncover the secrets of balanced nutrition. We'll also delve into the significance of staying hydrated and the art of portion control. With this knowledge, you'll be equipped to make informed dietary choices, promoting overall well-being and a harmonious relationship with food.

Macronutrients: The Building Blocks of the Body

Macronutrients are essential components of our diet, including proteins, carbohydrates, and fats. They provide the body with energy and support various physiological functions.

Proteins are the essential building blocks for both growth and repair, functioning much like diligent construction workers within our bodies. They are particularly vital for children and teenagers, who are undergoing rapid developmental phases, as proteins aid in forming tissues such as muscles, bones, and organs. Beyond mere growth, proteins are integral to the body's repair processes, healing wounds and mending muscle strains to reinforce our overall strength.

These proteins are composed of amino acids, which are the basic units that combine to create a wide array of proteins, each with its distinct role. Our diet is the primary source of these amino acids, underscoring the significance of a varied protein-rich diet that includes meat, fish, eggs, dairy, beans, and nuts. Such dietary diversity ensures we obtain all the necessary amino acids for the effective upkeep and maintenance of our bodies.

Carbohydrates serve as the primary energy source for our bodies, akin to fuel in an engine. They are predominantly found in foods like bread, rice, pasta, fruits, and vegetables. During digestion, carbohydrates are broken down into glucose, which powers brain function and muscle movement. Our bodies also store carbohydrates as glycogen in the liver and muscles, acting as a reserve energy source. However, it's crucial to differentiate between simple and complex carbohydrates.

Simple carbohydrates, often referred to as simple sugars, consist of one or two sugar molecules, making them easily and quickly digestible by the body. They provide a rapid source of energy, but this quick energy spike can lead to a subsequent crash, which is why they are sometimes labeled as 'bad'. However, not all simple carbohydrates are harmful. Fruits, for example, contain natural simple sugars but also offer essential nutrients and fiber, making them a healthy choice. On the other hand, processed and refined sugars found in sodas, candies, and baked goods lack nutritional value and contribute to weight gain and other health issues, hence are considered 'bad' simple carbohydrates.

Complex carbohydrates, in contrast, are composed of longer chains of sugar molecules, which take longer for the body to break down. This results in a more gradual release of energy, making them more beneficial for sustained energy levels. Examples of healthy complex carbohydrates include whole grains, brown rice, legumes, and starchy vegetables, which are not only energy-rich but also packed with fiber, vitamins, and minerals. However, not all complex carbs are equally beneficial. Refined grains, like white bread and white pasta, have been stripped of their nutritional value during processing, rendering them 'bad' complex carbohydrates. These refined grains can cause rapid spikes in blood sugar and contribute to weight gain and other health issues, similar to 'bad' simple carbohydrates.

Dietary fiber, an integral part of carbohydrates, plays multiple roles in maintaining health. It aids digestion, manages blood sugar levels, reduces bad cholesterol, and assists in weight management. Fiber-rich foods include whole grains, fruits, and vegetables, essential for a balanced diet.

Fats, or lipids, are misunderstood but essential macronutrients. They store energy, aid in absorbing fat-soluble vitamins, contribute to cell structure, and are vital for brain health. Omega-3 and omega-6 fatty acids, in particular, are crucial for cognitive functions. While moderation is key, healthy fats from avocados, nuts, and olive oil are important for well-being.

Micronutrients: Essential Vitamins and Minerals

Vitamins and minerals are indispensable micronutrients that play pivotal roles in maintaining our health and well-being. Vitamins, essential for various biochemical processes, serve as coenzymes or cofactors in enzymatic reactions, support the immune system, and act as antioxidants. For instance, Vitamin C aids in collagen production, crucial for skin, bones, and blood vessels, while vitamins A and D are vital for eye health and bone strength, respectively. Antioxidants like vitamins E and C protect cells from damage by free radicals, thereby preventing chronic diseases.

Minerals, distinct from vitamins as inorganic elements, are categorized into major and trace minerals. Major minerals, including calcium and potassium, are necessary in larger amounts for functions like building bones, muscle function, and regulating blood pressure. Trace minerals, such as iron, zinc, and selenium, though needed in smaller quantities, are vital for oxygen transport, immune function, and cellular protection.

Micronutrient-rich foods are central to acquiring these nutrients. Fruits and vegetables provide vitamins like C and A and minerals like potassium. Whole grains offer B vitamins and essential minerals like iron and magnesium. Nuts and seeds are sources of minerals like selenium and copper, along with vitamin E. Dairy products supply calcium and vitamin D, crucial for bone health, while lean meats, poultry, and fish are rich in iron, zinc, and selenium.

Understanding the two main categories of vitamins – fat-soluble (A, D, E, K) and water-soluble (C and B vitamins) – is essential for dietary planning. Fat-soluble vitamins, stored in body fat, require careful intake to avoid toxicity, while water-soluble vitamins, not readily stored, necessitate regular consumption to avoid deficiencies.

Deficiencies in these micronutrients can have significant health impacts. Vitamin D deficiency, for instance, can lead to weakened bones, while lack of vitamin C can cause scurvy. Vitamin A deficiency is linked to night blindness, and B12 deficiency can result in anemia and nerve damage. A balanced diet is crucial for preventing these deficiencies.

Balancing micronutrient intake involves a diverse diet, mindful portion sizes, and awareness of nutrient interactions. For example, calcium and magnesium aid each other's absorption, while excessive calcium can inhibit iron absorption. Dietary restrictions and health conditions may necessitate special attention to certain micronutrients. Consulting a healthcare professional for personalized guidance is advisable for specific dietary needs.

A well-rounded diet rich in various foods is key to obtaining essential vitamins and minerals. These micronutrients support numerous vital functions in the body, from bone health and immune function to cell protection and energy production. Balancing their intake is essential for maintaining optimal health and preventing nutrient deficiencies.

Daily Nutritional Needs

Our bodies rely on a variety of nutrients to function optimally, and striking the right balance of these nutrients is key to overall health. These nutrients serve as the building blocks for growth, repair, and energy production in the body.

Caloric intake is fundamental to our nutrition, acting as the fuel that powers all bodily functions, ranging from the basal metabolic rate (the energy required to keep the body functioning at rest) to the energy expended during physical activities. The number of calories an individual requires can vary greatly, influenced by factors such as age, gender, activity level, and metabolic efficiency. To illustrate this variation, consider a few examples:

- A sedentary adult woman typically requires about 1,600 to 2,000 calories per day to maintain her weight, while a sedentary adult man might need about 2,000 to 2,600 calories. These values can fluctuate based on age, with younger adults generally requiring more calories.

- For those who are more active, the caloric needs increase. An adult woman with a moderately active lifestyle may need between 1,800 and 2,200 calories daily, whereas a moderately active adult man might require 2,200 to 2,800 calories.

- Athletes or individuals with very active lifestyles may need even more calories. For instance, a highly active woman could require 2,000 to 2,400 calories daily, while a similarly active man might need between 2,400 and 3,000 calories.

It's important to emphasize that these are approximate values and individual needs can vary significantly. Balancing calorie intake with physical activity is crucial for maintaining a healthy weight. Consuming more calories than the body burns can lead to weight gain, while consuming too few can lead to weight loss and potential nutrient deficiencies. Therefore, understanding one's personal caloric needs and adjusting intake accordingly, possibly with the guidance of a healthcare professional or a registered dietitian, is essential for optimal health and well-being.

Nearly everything we consume, from food to beverages, contributes to our daily caloric intake, with a few exceptions like water. Within these calories, macronutrients — carbohydrates, proteins, and fats — are fundamental, each playing a unique and essential role in our health..

In addition to macronutrients, micronutrients, although required in smaller quantities, are equally important. A diet rich in fruits, vegetables, whole grains, and lean proteins is typically adequate to meet these micronutrient needs, ensuring a comprehensive nutritional profile.

Fiber, a specific type of carbohydrate, deserves special attention due to its role in digestive health. The recommended daily intake of fiber for adults is about 25 to 30 grams. This can be met by incorporating a variety of fiber-rich foods into the diet, such as whole grains, fruits, and vegetables.

As a general guideline, strive to consume approximately 1 gram of protein per pound of your desired body weight. Furthermore, when planning meals, aim to fill at least half of your plate with vegetables. Prioritize water as your primary beverage, and incorporate fermented foods and healthy fats into your daily diet.

For personalized caloric guidance that reflects your unique needs based on age, activity level, and other individual factors, delving into the Recommended Daily Allowances (RDAs) can be highly beneficial. These allowances, established by health authorities, provide guidelines for essential nutrient intake tailored to various demographics. RDAs differ across nutrients, taking into account specific variables such as age, gender, and life stage. By following these recommendations, individuals can make well-informed dietary decisions that contribute to maintaining their overall health and well-being.

Hydration

Our bodies, likened to complex machines, rely on water as their vital fuel. About 60% of our body is water, present in our blood, muscles, and bones. This liquid is crucial for transporting nutrients and oxygen to cells, energy production, and overall functioning. Inadequate hydration can result in fatigue and decreased performance.

Water also helps regulate body temperature. When overheated, we sweat to cool down, and sweat's evaporation from the skin lowers body temperature. Insufficient water intake can hinder this cooling process, posing risks of overheating, particularly in hot conditions or during physical activities. Additionally, water is vital for digestion, aiding in food breakdown and nutrient absorption. A lack of hydration can lead to digestive issues like constipation and joint discomfort due to inadequate lubrication.

Moreover, our brain's function depends heavily on water. Dehydration can impair cognitive abilities, causing concentration difficulties, memory issues, and mood swings. Therefore, staying hydrated is crucial for mental sharpness and alertness. Hydration also impacts our skin and appearance, with well-hydrated skin appearing healthier and more radiant, while dehydration can lead to dryness and premature aging.

Understanding your daily water needs is vital, as these vary depending on climate, physical activity, and individual body size. Hot and humid climates increase sweating, requiring more water intake, whereas cooler climates might reduce these needs. Physical activity levels also influence hydration needs, with increased sweating during activities necessitating more water intake. Additionally, larger individuals or those with different metabolic rates, like children and the elderly, may have varied hydration requirements.

A good rule of thumb, as proposed by Dr Mark Hyman, is to drink half your weight (in pounds) in ounces of water. So if you weigh 100 pounds, you should drink around 50 ounces of water a day.

For those of us on the metric system, it converts to drinking 33 milliliters of water for every kilogram of weight. So if you weigh 45 kilograms then you should drink 1 and a half liters of water a day.

However, this is a basic guideline and doesn't take into account variables such as climate and exertion levels. Listening to your body is key; thirst is a natural indicator of needing water.

Dehydration, the condition of insufficient bodily water, has signs like thirst, dark yellow urine, dry mouth, and dry skin. Severe dehydration can lead to dizziness, rapid heartbeat, low blood pressure, and even heat-related illnesses, which are medical emergencies. Cognitive function can also be affected, impacting concentration and mood. Particular attention should be given to vulnerable groups like the elderly and children, who might not easily recognize dehydration signs.

Conversely, overhydration or hyponatremia, resulting from excessive water intake, can lead to sodium level dilution in the bloodstream. Symptoms include nausea, headache, confusion, and in severe cases, seizures or coma. This condition is particularly relevant for endurance athletes, who may drink more than what is lost through sweating. To prevent this, it's important to balance water and electrolyte intake.

Electrolytes, like sodium and potassium, play a crucial role in hydration and bodily functions. They help regulate fluid balance and are essential for muscle and nerve function. Foods rich in these electrolytes, such as bananas, spinach, and yogurt, can help maintain a healthy balance, especially during exercise.

To stay hydrated, it's beneficial to listen to your body, carry a water bottle, set drinking reminders, and flavor your water if needed. Adjusting fluid intake according to the environment and physical activity is also important, as is choosing foods with high water content.

Portion Control: Finding the Right Balance

Portion control involves managing the amount of food consumed during meals and snacks. This is a simple concept with significant health impacts. By controlling portion sizes, we can manage calorie intake and prevent excess energy storage as fat, aiding in weight maintenance. It also ensures a balanced nutrient intake, preventing overindulgence in specific food types and ensuring a well-rounded mix of vitamins, minerals, and proteins.

Grasping the concept of portion control is essential for making informed dietary choices, and this can be achieved through several methods. Firstly, adhering to food label recommendations provides a clear guideline for appropriate serving sizes. Additionally, employing the "handy" method offers a practical and visual guide: estimate protein servings using the size of your palm, a clenched fist for vegetable portions, a cupped hand for carbohydrates, and your thumb for fats.

Central to effective portion control is the practice of mindful eating, which encompasses both being fully present and attentive during meals and tuning into your body's signals of hunger and fullness. This approach aids in recognizing when you are truly hungry or satisfied, thus preventing overeating.

Consuming nutrient-dense foods is also helpful for portion control as these foods offer essential nutrients without an overload of calories. Typically, these are whole foods, including a variety of leafy greens, fruits such as berries and apples, lean protein sources like fish and beans, whole grains such as quinoa, along with nuts, seeds, and dairy or wholesome plant-based alternatives.

Finally, employ visual cues. Utilizing smaller plates can give the illusion of larger servings, helping to satisfy visual hunger cues. Additionally, a vibrant array of colors on your plate often signifies a diversity of nutrients, contributing to a well-rounded diet. Strategically dividing your plate into specific sections for various food groups can further ensure a balanced and nutrient-rich meal, promoting a holistic approach to healthy eating.

FAD DIET DILEMMAS

Dieting has become a major part of modern culture, influenced by psychological factors, societal norms, and the desire for quick fixes. In this exploration, we aim to understand why dieting is so popular, examining its appeal from the promise of fast results to societal body image ideals, and the role of media and celebrities in promoting these trends. By the end of this, you should have a clearer understanding of both the allure and the potential downsides and limitations of dieting.

Why Dieting is Popular

The popularity of dieting in contemporary society can be attributed to a vast number of psychological, social, and cultural factors. Many are attracted to diets because of their longing for immediate results. Fad diets, offering quick weight loss, appeal to those craving swift solutions. Societal pressures to conform to certain beauty standards, amplified by media and advertising showcasing idealized body images, contribute to body dissatisfaction and the pursuit of these regimens. Emotional factors like stress, anxiety, and a desire for control over eating habits are additional motivators.

Social pressures and trends, heavily influenced by social media, further explain dieting's popularity. Platforms like Instagram and TikTok have become arenas where influencers and celebrities promote various diets, creating a sense of urgency to follow these trends. Peer pressure and cultural norms valuing thinness also play significant roles, pushing individuals towards dieting to fit in and be accepted. The weight loss industry capitalizes on these trends with aggressive marketing, perpetuating the cycle.

Celebrity endorsements significantly impact these fad trends also. When public figures promote diets and share their success stories, it creates a compelling narrative for fans and followers. This influence is especially pronounced among adolescents and teenagers, who view celebrities as role models and may emulate their eating behaviors without fully understanding the potential risks.

In essence, the popularity of dieting is fueled by a blend of psychological desires, societal influences, celebrity endorsements, and the seductive appeal of quick results. While these factors make dieting appealing, it's vital to approach weight loss with a focus on long-term health and sustainable habits rather than temporary solutions.

Why Dieting Doesn't Work

One major reason diets don't work is due to the way our body reacts to them. Often, diets emphasize extreme restrictions on certain food groups and overconsumption of others, leading to nutrient deficiencies and an unbalanced intake of vitamins, minerals, and other vital components. This can result in fatigue, poor health, and a slowed metabolism that conserves energy and retains fat, making it harder to lose weight in the long run.

Additionally, such diets often trigger cravings and binge-eating episodes, undermining the efforts of dieting in the first place. Unrealistic restrictions, like extreme calorie cutting or eliminating entire food groups, are not sustainable and may lead to rapid weight regain once regular eating habits resume. These diets also fail to consider individual factors such as age, gender, activity level, metabolism, and genetic makeup, making them ineffective for many people.

Metabolic adaptation is another critical factor. As the body adapts to reduced calorie intake by slowing down the metabolism and breaking down muscle for energy, it becomes harder to lose weight and easier to regain it. This leads to the "Yo-Yo Effect," where rapid weight loss followed by weight regain creates a frustrating cycle of repeated dieting attempts with limited success.

The emotional toll of dieting cannot be overlooked either. Strict diets often lead to frustration, guilt, anxiety, low self-esteem, and a disrupted connection with natural hunger cues. This negative relationship with food complicates long-term adherence.

All these factors and more collectively underscore the importance of a more balanced, sustainable, and personalized approach to eating for long-term health and weight management success.

The Solution: Dieting vs. Lifestyle Change

Balanced nutrition is vital in preventing nutritional deficiencies, characterized by a lack of essential nutrients like vitamins, minerals, and proteins. These deficiencies can lead to various health problems and reduced energy levels. A balanced diet, incorporating a variety of foods from all food groups such as fruits, vegetables, grains, proteins, and dairy, ensures we get the necessary mix of nutrients.

Key benefits of balanced nutrition include maintaining a healthy weight and supporting the immune system. Focusing on whole, nutrient-dense foods over empty calories helps control calorie intake and prevent weight gain. Nutrients like vitamin C, found in fruits and vegetables, are crucial for a strong immune system. Additionally, a balanced diet contributes to better digestion and gut health. Fiber-rich foods like whole grains and vegetables support regular bowel movements and a healthy gut microbiome.

Improving your relationship with food is crucial for lasting dietary changes. Unlike fad diets that focus on restrictions and labeling foods as "good" or "bad," a positive approach views food as nourishment. This mindset avoids guilt and shame associated with eating and embraces moderation. Lifestyle changes, rather than strict diets, advocate a balanced approach to eating, reducing anxiety and stress. This includes listening to your body's hunger and fullness cues and practicing mindful eating to enjoy meals fully.

In contrast to fad diets that offer quick fixes but are hard to maintain, lifestyle changes involve creating sustainable habits. These gradual adjustments in eating patterns and routines are more manageable in the long run, avoiding the yo-yo dieting cycle of weight loss and regain. This approach promotes steady progress and prioritizes a balanced, nutritious diet for overall well-being.

Embracing gradual progress is key in transitioning from fad diets to lifestyle changes. Rather than demanding significant changes at once, a gradual approach allows for manageable changes over time. This reduces the overwhelming feeling and supports learning and adapting to new eating habits and routines.

Considering the social impact of restrictive dietary choices is also important. Fad diets' strict rules can make social gatherings challenging, potentially leading to isolation. Lifestyle changes offer more flexibility, allowing for balanced choices in social settings and open communication about dietary goals with friends and family. This support network is essential for staying on track and enjoying social events without diet-related stress.

Navigating the complex world of dieting, it's clear that quick fixes and drastic changes often eclipse essential aspects of nutrition and mental health. This calls for a change from temporary, restrictive diets to a holistic approach that values long-term health, sustainable eating, and a healthy attitude towards food. Acknowledging that dietary needs vary, emotional health matters, and mindful eating is beneficial leads to a more balanced, satisfying way of life. Moving from short-term diets to a broader, lifestyle-focused view on nutrition is key to real, enduring wellness and a healthier society.

GROCERY SHOPPING

In this section we will dive into the multifaceted aspects of grocery shopping - from developing a health-centric shopping list, understanding the nuances of nutritional labels, and mastering budget-friendly strategies, to making sustainable and ethical choices. These elements are crucial not just for personal well-being but also for the larger good of society and the planet.

Creating a Healthy Shopping List

Creating a shopping list offers numerous advantages for a more efficient, cost-effective, and healthier grocery shopping experience. The primary benefit is improved organization. With a list, you're less likely to forget essential items, more likely to adhere to your budget, and can avoid aimless wandering that leads to impulse buys and overspending. This methodical approach is especially beneficial for busy individuals or families with hectic schedules.

Planning meals and snacks in advance and noting the required ingredients on your list encourages the purchase of nutritious foods. This focus on healthy choices is particularly advantageous for those maintaining a balanced diet or managing specific health conditions, as it aligns with dietary goals. In contrast, ultra-processed foods, often found in bright packaging with long ingredient lists, are less desirable. They typically contain high levels of added sugars, unhealthy fats, and artificial additives. To make healthier choices, prioritize fresh foods like fruits, vegetables, and lean proteins, which are packed with essential nutrients, vitamins, and minerals. When purchasing packaged foods, carefully read labels to avoid added sugars, trans fats, and excessive sodium.

Another advantage of using a shopping list is time efficiency. Knowing exactly what you need reduces time spent in store aisles, a valuable aspect for those with limited time. This method also contributes to reducing food waste, as buying only what you need means fewer perishable items are left unused and discarded. This not only saves money but also promotes a sustainable approach to food consumption.

Lastly, a well-thought-out shopping list can enhance the overall experience by reducing stress. It provides a sense of control and confidence, minimizing the anxiety of forgetting something important or making hasty decisions.

Understanding Nutritional Labels

Nutritional labels on food products serve as essential guides, helping us make informed choices about what we consume. These labels not only reveal the calorie content of food items, essential for managing weight and maintaining a balanced diet, but also provide detailed information about the nutrients present, such as fats, carbohydrates, proteins, vitamins, and minerals. This is particularly beneficial for individuals with specific dietary needs, like those with diabetes or food allergies, enabling them to avoid foods that might cause health issues.

A key component of these labels is the serving size, which forms the basis for all the nutritional information provided. It's crucial to adjust the values on the label according to the actual amount consumed, as the listed calories and nutrients correspond to this specified serving size. The "Servings per Container" tells you how many servings are in the entire package, further aiding in managing intake.

The calorie content and its distribution across different categories like fats, carbohydrates, and proteins are central to these labels. Not all calories are equal; some, like fats and sugars, may offer less nutritional value. Hence, it's vital to consider both the total calorie count and its sources.

Added sugars and sugar alcohols are other important elements on these labels. Added sugars are those not naturally occurring in food and should be limited due to their potential health risks. Sugar alcohols, used in sugar-free or reduced-sugar products, offer an alternative sweetness but might lead to digestive issues in some individuals.

Lastly, the Percent Daily Value (%DV) is a crucial aspect, indicating how much a serving of food contributes to your daily nutritional needs, usually based on a 2,000-calorie diet. This helps in comparing products and aligning food choices with dietary preferences and requirements.

Nutritional labels are vital tools in promoting healthy eating habits, enabling product comparisons, and increasing awareness about nutrition. By understanding these labels, we can make choices that support our health and well-being, fostering a more mindful approach to our diet.

Budget-Friendly Shopping Tips

When it comes to grocery shopping, setting a budget is a fundamental step to manage your finances wisely. By determining how much you're willing to spend on groceries within a certain period, like a week or a month, you can avoid overspending and financial strain. Start by analyzing your income and expenses to gauge your disposable income. This will guide you in deciding how much to allocate for groceries, considering factors like family size and dietary needs.

Be realistic when setting your budget. A larger family or special dietary requirements may necessitate a higher budget, while singles or smaller households might manage with less. To adhere to your budget, track your spending, and make use of grocery lists and mobile apps.

Remember, a budget doesn't mean sacrificing quality or nutrition. It's about informed choices and spending mindfulness. Comparing prices is also vital. Look at the price per unit, compare different brands, and use a grocery list to identify the best deals. Keep an eye out for sales, discounts, and coupons to further stretch your budget. Coupons, whether from newspapers or digital sources, can offer considerable savings, especially when combined with sales. Joining store loyalty programs and keeping track of store flyers and circulars are other effective strategies.

Buying non-perishable items in bulk, especially those you frequently use, can be cost-effective. This reduces shopping frequency and impulse buys, though it requires mindful storage and expiration date monitoring. Similarly, opting for generic or store-brand products instead of name brands can lead to significant savings without quality compromise.

Another practical tip is to avoid shopping when hungry, as this can lead to impulsive purchases and budget overruns. Planning your trips post-meal or having a snack beforehand can be greatly beneficial. Finally, consider buying frozen and canned produce, which often offer better affordability and longer shelf life than fresh produce, without significantly compromising on nutritional value.

Sustainable and Ethical Choices

Making sustainable and ethical choices in our grocery purchases can significantly contribute to a healthier planet and a more equitable society, ensuring a better future for all.

Sustainability in grocery shopping entails choosing items that minimize waste, reduce carbon emissions, and protect ecosystems. For example, buying locally grown produce not only supports local economies but also lowers transportation emissions, helping to combat climate change. Opting for products with minimal packaging, especially those avoiding single-use plastics, reduces the amount of waste in landfills and oceans.

Ethical shopping extends beyond environmental considerations, focusing on the welfare of people and animals involved in the food production process. It involves being mindful of fair labor practices, ensuring workers are paid fairly and work in safe conditions. It also means supporting brands that prioritize humane treatment of animals and responsible sourcing.

Another crucial aspect of ethical shopping is understanding and recognizing ethical label certifications, like Fair Trade and USDA Organic. These labels guide consumers toward products meeting specific ethical and sustainable standards, ensuring that their purchases align with their values.

Reducing food waste is also important. Careful meal planning, paying attention to expiration dates, proper food storage, and creative use of leftovers can minimize the amount of food wasted. Composting is another effective way to manage food scraps, turning them into nutrient-rich soil.

Conscious consumerism involves being informed about the products we buy, supporting brands that prioritize sustainability, and considering the longevity and durability of products. Conscious consumerism also means being aware of the social and ethical implications of purchases and choosing items that reflect one's values and beliefs.

By making sustainable and ethical choices in our grocery shopping, we send a message to producers and retailers that we value environmentally friendly and socially responsible products. As consumer demand shifts towards these values, companies are incentivized to adopt more sustainable and ethical practices, leading to a more just and eco-friendly food industry. Our everyday choices have the power to make a positive impact on the world, contributing to a sustainable and ethical future.

MEAL PLANNING AND PREPARATION

The idea of meal prepping and preparation combines nutrition, efficiency, savings, and even social connections in daily life. It's a blend of planning, creativity, and execution that fits busy schedules with healthy meals.

The Benefits of Meal Planning

Meal planning stands out as a practical approach to enhancing our daily lives, offering a wide range of benefits from healthier eating choices to social connections. This method of organizing meals in advance empowers individuals and families to actively manage their diet, leading to better nutrition and overall well-being.

One of the key advantages of meal planning is the emphasis on healthy eating. By planning meals, you can thoughtfully select ingredients, prioritizing fresh fruits, vegetables, lean proteins, and whole grains. These nutrient-rich options are packed with essential vitamins and minerals, promoting optimal health. Meal planning also aids in avoiding unhealthy temptations and convenience foods, which are often less nutritious. This proactive approach to diet ensures that each meal contributes positively to your health goals.

Another significant benefit is the practice of portion control, a vital aspect of maintaining a balanced diet. Meal planning allows for pre-determined serving sizes, preventing overeating and helping to manage weight. This is especially crucial for those with dietary restrictions or health conditions such as diabetes, as consistent meal sizes help regulate blood sugar levels. Furthermore, mindful portion sizes enhance the dining experience, allowing for a greater appreciation of food's flavors and textures.

Financial savings are an often-overlooked advantage of meal planning. By creating a detailed shopping list and sticking to it, impulse buys are reduced, leading to lower grocery bills. Bulk buying and taking advantage of sales further add to the cost-effectiveness. Additionally, meal planning reduces food waste, aligning with both budget-friendly and environmentally sustainable practices.

Time efficiency is another key aspect of meal planning. With a clear plan in place, decision-making is streamlined, and grocery shopping becomes more efficient. Batch cooking or using methods like slow cooking can save considerable time, allowing for a more relaxed and manageable schedule.

Beyond personal benefits, meal planning fosters social and familial connections. It encourages shared responsibilities and teamwork within the family, turning meal preparation into a collaborative effort. Regular family meals, a result of organized planning, become opportunities for meaningful interactions and stronger relationships. Additionally, meal planning facilitates social gatherings, making hosting and entertaining more feasible and enjoyable.

Meal planning is a holistic approach that positively impacts various aspects of life. It promotes health through nutrient-rich meals and portion control, saves time and money, and strengthens family and social bonds. By incorporating meal planning into your routine, you can enjoy a healthier, more organized, and socially enriched lifestyle.

Creating a Healthy Meal Plan

Creating a balanced meal plan is essential for maintaining overall health and achieving specific dietary goals. Whether you're aiming for weight management, muscle gain, or simply want to improve your well-being, a well-structured meal plan can make a significant difference.

Here are some recommended steps you can take to create a balanced meal plan tailored to your needs and preferences:

1. Begin by determining your dietary objectives, taking into account any dietary restrictions or preferences you may have, such as vegetarianism or gluten-free choices.

2. Estimate your daily calorie requirements using a reliable online calculator or by consulting a nutritionist. Factors like age, gender, activity level, and your specific goals will influence this calculation.

3. Divide your daily calorie allowance into three main meals (breakfast, lunch, and dinner) and, if needed, two snacks. This division helps in managing hunger and energy levels throughout the day.

4. Calculate your protein needs. Aim to consume approximately 1 gram of protein per pound of your target body weight each day. This helps in building and repairing tissues, especially if you are working towards muscle gain.

5. Fill at least half of your plate with vegetables (fruits count here too). Variety is beneficial; however, if you find it challenging to eat a wide range of vegetables, start by choosing the ones you like and gradually branch out to others.

6. Make sure to incorporate fermented foods like Greek yogurt or kimchi, as well as healthy fats into your daily diet. These contribute to gut health and overall well-being.

7. Once you know your main ingredients, you can decide exactly what you want to cook. Look online for recipes and adjust them to suit your needs.

Remember to periodically reassess and adjust your meal plan based on your progress and how you feel. A flexible approach allows you to make changes as your body and lifestyle evolve.

Healthy Cooking Tips

Balancing flavor and nutrition is an essential aspect of meal planning and preparation, leading to delicious, satisfying, and healthy meals. Using a variety of ingredients and cooking methods is key. Incorporating fruits, vegetables, lean proteins, and whole grains adds diversity and essential nutrients. Cooking techniques like grilling, roasting, steaming, or sautéing enhance natural flavors.

Herbs and spices play a crucial role in creating meals that are both tasty and nutritious, without relying on excess salt, sugar, or unhealthy fats. Portion control is also crucial when cooking. Often, people tend to eat what is prepared, even if they are not hungry. Prevent this by only cooking what you need. It can take a bit of practice to adjust to this, but it's worth the effort. Enjoyment of food is also an important aspect, as adjusting recipes to personal tastes encourages adherence to a healthy eating plan.

Healthy cooking methods such as steaming, baking, roasting, and grilling are essential. Steaming retains nutrients better than boiling. Baking or roasting requires little to no added fats, and grilling allows excess fats to drip away. Sautéing in a small amount of healthy oil preserves flavor and texture, while boiling is excellent for grains and soups when done correctly.

Choosing the right cooking oil impacts flavor and nutritional value. Healthy options include extra virgin olive oil, avocado oil, coconut oil, and grass-fed ghee. Each has unique benefits and uses, suitable for different cooking methods and health considerations. Be cautious with fats that can be unhealthy; some margarines, certain types of palm oil, and various vegetable oils may contain unhealthy trans fats.

Smart ingredient substitutions can make dishes healthier. Greek yogurt, for instance, can replace sour cream or mayonnaise; unsweetened applesauce or mashed bananas can substitute for butter or oil in baking; and lean poultry can be used instead of ground beef. Natural sweeteners like honey or maple syrup can replace refined sugar, and herbs and spices can reduce sodium intake. Whole wheat or whole-grain pasta is a healthier alternative to regular pasta.

Incorporating vegetable-centric dishes is another smart, nutritious choice. Salads, stir-fries, roasted vegetables, soups, stews, and vegetable-infused pasta dishes add essential vitamins, minerals, and dietary fiber.

Food safety is paramount in meal preparation. Firstly, proper hygiene is essential. This means washing your hands with soap and water before and after handling food, which helps prevent the spread of harmful bacteria that can make us sick. Also, make sure your cooking utensils and cutting boards are clean.

Preventing cross-contamination is another crucial aspect of food safety. Keep raw meat, poultry, and seafood separate from other foods, especially fruits and vegetables. Bacteria from these raw foods can easily transfer to other items, so it's important to use separate cutting boards and utensils when working with them.

Cooking to safe temperatures is a must. Different types of foods need to reach specific temperatures to kill harmful bacteria. For example, chicken should be cooked to an internal temperature of 165°F (74°C) to ensure it's safe to eat. Using a food thermometer can help you check if your food has reached the right temperature.

Prompt refrigeration is also vital. After cooking or buying perishable foods like meat, dairy, or leftovers, it's important to refrigerate them within two hours. Keeping foods at a temperature below 40°F (4°C) slows down the growth of harmful bacteria, which can spoil food and make it unsafe to eat.

Checking expiration dates is another key step in food safety. Finally, employing safe defrosting methods is crucial. If you need to thaw frozen food, it's best to do it in the refrigerator, in cold water, or in the microwave. Avoid leaving food out at room temperature to thaw, as this can promote the growth of bacteria.

Batch Cooking

Batch cooking is the practice of preparing meals in large quantities. By dedicating a block of time to cook and store multiple servings, you not only save time on busy days but also reduce the temptation to opt for less healthy fast food or takeout.

Economically, buying ingredients in bulk often results in discounts and less food waste, which in turn decreases grocery bills. This method of cooking allows for more control over ingredients, aiding in healthier meal choices free of excessive additives and preservatives found in convenience foods.

Additionally, batch cooking encourages experimentation with recipes and contributes to environmental sustainability by reducing the reliance on single-use food packaging.

To optimize the batch cooking process, certain kitchen tools are indispensable. Airtight storage containers are essential for keeping food fresh and preventing spoilage. A variety of sharp knives facilitates efficient ingredient preparation, while a large stockpot or Dutch oven is ideal for soups, stews, and sauces. A slow cooker simplifies meal preparation with minimal effort, and a food processor or blender can speed up chopping and blending tasks. Lastly, having an array of baking sheets and casserole dishes accommodates different meal types and quantities.

Adapting recipes for batch cooking requires a bit of practice, but by making adjustments to the ingredients and cooking times, you can create delicious and efficient meals that fit your meal plan perfectly.

Let's start with ingredient quantities. When you're making a larger batch, you typically need more of all the ingredients. For instance, if a recipe calls for 2 cups of flour, you may need 4 cups to double it. However, it's important to exercise caution with spices and seasonings – you don't always need to double them. Instead, it's a better approach to add them gradually and taste the food as you go to ensure you don't overdo it.

Additionally, you might need to tweak the cooking times and temperatures. Cooking a larger batch can take more time for everything to cook evenly. Therefore, you might have to increase the cooking time or slightly lower the temperature to prevent the outside from burning while the inside remains undercooked. Keeping a close eye on your food and using a thermometer if you're uncertain about its readiness is a good practice.

Proper storage is a key factor in keeping your meals safe and delicious. Before freezing your cooked dishes, it's important to let them cool down first. This prevents condensation from forming inside the containers, which can lead to freezer burn. Once your meals have cooled, it's time to pack them up. Using airtight containers or freezer-safe bags is essential. These containers keep your food protected from freezer odors and help maintain its quality.

Labeling your containers is another important step. Write down the preparation date and the contents of each container. This way, you'll always know how long your meals have been in the freezer and what's inside. It's a simple practice that can save you from unpleasant surprises later on. If you're cooking in large quantities, consider dividing your meals into smaller portions before freezing. This makes it easier to take out just what you need when it's time to reheat.

For extra protection, you can use a vacuum sealer. It removes air from the containers, further preventing freezer burn and extending the shelf life of your batch-cooked meals. However, it's not always necessary for every dish, so consider whether it's worth the extra step for your specific recipes.

Thawing is another crucial aspect of batch cooking. The safest way to thaw your frozen meals is in the refrigerator. This slow and gentle method prevents bacterial growth and maintains the texture and flavor of your food. Plan ahead and give your meals enough time to thaw, as it can take several hours or even overnight, depending on the size of the dish. Avoid thawing at room temperature, as it can lead to unsafe temperatures and compromise the quality of your food.

MANAGING EMOTIONAL EATING

Emotional eating is a common challenge, driven by a mix of psychological and emotional factors, often leading to eating based on emotions rather than hunger. Understanding this behavior involves gaining insights into our eating patterns and recognizing the emotional triggers that drive us to eat. In this section we uncover its layers, from triggers to healthier coping strategies, providing a comprehensive perspective on managing this aspect of our relationship with food.

The Emotional Eating Cycle

Emotional eating often adheres to a predictable seven-stage cycle, key to both understanding and managing the behavior.

The cycle begins with an emotional trigger, such as stress, sadness, anger, or boredom, which prompts a person to turn to food for solace. These emotions serve as the spark for the ensuing cycle. Following this, the emotional response stage occurs, where individuals react to their triggers in various ways, like anxiety or feeling overwhelmed.

The third stage is characterized by food cravings, intense desires for specific foods, usually comfort or junk foods, believed to alleviate emotional discomfort. This leads to the fourth stage, overeating, where the individual consumes more food than necessary or intended.

After overeating, the fifth stage is a temporary sense of relief. Eating distracts from emotional distress, offering short-lived comfort. However, this stage quickly gives way to guilt and shame, the sixth stage, where individuals regret their overindulgence and feel ashamed of their lack of control.

The final stage is the repetition of the cycle. The resurgence of emotional triggers leads to a return to food for coping, thus perpetuating the cycle.

In understanding these seven stages - emotional trigger, response, craving, overeating, relief, guilt, and repetition - individuals are better equipped to develop strategies and coping mechanisms to manage emotional eating. By recognizing each stage, it becomes possible to interrupt the cycle and address the underlying emotional triggers more effectively.

Identifying Your Emotional Triggers

Emotional triggers are essentially the events, thoughts, or feelings that prompt an individual to eat as a way to comfort themselves or distract from negative emotions. These triggers can be both external, like a stressful situation at work, and internal, such as feelings of sadness or anxiety.

Common emotional triggers include stress, boredom, loneliness, sadness, anxiety, and surprisingly, even happiness. For example, stress releases hormones like cortisol that increase cravings for high-calorie foods, while boredom or loneliness might lead to mindless eating as a form of entertainment or companionship. Positive emotions, like happiness during celebratory occasions, can also lead to indulgent eating as a form of reward.

To manage emotional eating effectively, it's crucial to distinguish between physical and emotional hunger. Physical hunger is a natural signal from the body indicating the need for nourishment, often accompanied by physical sensations like a growling stomach. In contrast, emotional hunger is sudden and driven by specific cravings, usually for comfort foods high in sugar and fat.

Identifying and understanding one's emotional triggers requires self-awareness and introspection. Techniques such as emotional journaling can be invaluable in this process. By keeping a record of thoughts, feelings, and eating circumstances, individuals can identify patterns and triggers behind their emotional eating habits. This journaling should include details like the time of day, emotions felt, and the types of food craved. Over time, this can reveal connections between certain emotions and eating behaviors.

Additionally, self-reflection plays a pivotal role in managing emotional eating. It involves asking oneself probing questions about current emotions and the desire to eat, examining eating patterns, and recognizing beliefs about food and emotions. This introspection can lead to the identification of healthier coping strategies, such as relaxation techniques, physical activities, or seeking support from friends, family, or professionals.

Developing Healthy Coping Mechanisms

Coping mechanisms play a crucial role in our lives, particularly in managing emotional eating. These mechanisms are our emotional safety nets, enabling us to navigate through challenging situations and make healthier choices. They are essential in handling stress, negative emotions, and building resilience, allowing us to face adversities without resorting to food as a crutch. By addressing the root causes of emotional eating, we can work towards sustainable solutions rather than relying on food as a temporary escape.

The development of emotional intelligence (EQ) is vital in this context. EQ involves understanding, managing, and effectively using emotions, both our own and others'. Recognizing and responding to our emotional states can prevent emotional eating. For instance, identifying stress or upset as triggers for overeating can lead to healthier coping strategies. Empathy, another EQ component, fosters connection and support, valuable in overcoming emotional eating. Additionally, regulating emotions through practices like relaxation techniques or seeking professional support helps in managing emotional eating.

Incorporating healthy distractions is another effective strategy. These activities provide alternative outlets for emotions and create a mental space between the urge to eat and actual eating, thus aiding in better control over emotional eating habits. Engaging in activities like walks, reading, or hobbies uplifts mood and enhances emotional well-being.

Effective stress management is also key. Techniques like deep breathing exercises, progressive muscle relaxation, mindfulness, meditation, and regular exercise can significantly reduce stress levels and the tendency to use food as a coping mechanism.

Social support is another cornerstone in managing emotional eating. Emotional comfort, practical assistance, accountability, and a sense of belonging provided by a robust support system are instrumental in overcoming emotional eating challenges.

Finally, seeking professional help is often crucial. Therapists and counselors bring expertise in addressing the psychological factors behind emotional eating. They provide a safe space for discussion and introduce evidence-based therapies like Cognitive-behavioral therapy (CBT), crucial in developing healthier coping mechanisms.

It's clear that emotional eating is a complex behavior that can lead to temporary comfort but lasting regrets. Managing it goes beyond merely changing eating habits; it involves self-awareness, emotional intelligence, and psychological resilience. By identifying emotional triggers and developing coping mechanisms, we can establish a healthier, more mindful relationship with food. This approach addresses both symptoms and root causes, fostering lasting change.

OVERCOMING FOOD CRAVINGS

Food cravings are not the same as basic hunger; they're complex reactions in our bodies. The goal is to understand the factors influencing cravings, from brain chemistry to daily routines, and make informed choices. When we understand why we crave certain foods, we can resist them and have a healthier and happier relationship with food.

Understanding Food Cravings

Delving into the science behind food cravings reveals a complex interplay of physiological, psychological, and environmental factors, going beyond mere lack of willpower. These intense desires for specific foods, often perceived as uncontrollable, stem from a variety of underlying causes.

Central to understanding cravings is the role of brain chemistry. Our brains seek pleasurable experiences, and certain foods, especially those high in sugar, fat, or salt, trigger the release of feel-good neurotransmitters like dopamine. This activation of the brain's reward system associates these foods with pleasure, leading to repeated cravings.

Hormones also significantly influence cravings. Ghrelin, the "hunger hormone," and leptin, the "satiety hormone," fluctuate to signal hunger and fullness, respectively. These fluctuations can intensify cravings, especially during periods of hunger.

Emotions and stress further complicate food cravings. Cortisol, a stress hormone, can increase cravings for comfort foods, making emotional eating a common coping mechanism. Additionally, our environment, including exposure to food-related cues like sights, smells, and advertisements, can trigger cravings, activating brain regions associated with reward and desire.

Nutrient deficiencies are another crucial aspect. Our bodies may crave specific foods as signals of lacking essential vitamins, minerals, or nutrients. For instance, iron deficiency might lead to cravings for red meat, while a lack of magnesium could trigger chocolate cravings. These deficiencies highlight the importance of a balanced diet in managing cravings.

Distinguishing between emotional eating and genuine cravings is vital. Emotional eating is driven by feelings and is not indicative of hunger, while cravings are intense desires for particular foods, arising from factors like nutrient deficiencies or hormonal imbalances. Recognizing this distinction is key to developing effective strategies for overcoming them.

Habitual cravings, linked to our routines and behaviors, also play a role. Daily rituals, such as having a sugary snack while watching TV, can create a habit of craving these items in specific contexts. Understanding these habitual cravings can help in breaking the cycle and making healthier choices.

The connection between cravings and sleep is another critical factor. Sleep deprivation disrupts hormonal balance, leading to increased appetite and cravings for high-calorie foods. This relationship is bidirectional, as consuming certain foods can disrupt sleep patterns, creating a cycle of poor sleep and increased cravings.

Common Triggers for Food Cravings

Although there are many triggers for food cravings, here we will just touch on 10 of the more common ones.

Low blood sugar, or hypoglycemia, is a key trigger for food cravings. When blood sugar levels fall, the body signals the brain for energy, often resulting in a strong desire for sugary or high-carbohydrate foods. This response is primarily because the brain, which heavily relies on glucose from carbohydrates, seeks a quick energy fix under low blood sugar conditions. Skipping meals or prolonged periods without eating can exacerbate this, as the body lacks a steady supply of nutrients, leading to hunger and cravings for energy-boosting foods.

Additionally, excessive intake of refined sugars and simple carbohydrates can cause a rapid spike and crash in blood sugar levels, further fueling cravings. It's crucial to manage blood sugar through balanced meals and snacks to prevent unhealthy eating habits and potential weight gain.

Pregnancy introduces another dimension to food cravings due to hormonal changes. Hormones like human chorionic gonadotropin (hCG), progesterone, and estrogen can influence a pregnant woman's sense of smell and taste, leading to specific food cravings. These hormonal fluctuations can also cause blood sugar level changes, prompting cravings for sweet or carbohydrate-rich foods. Understanding and indulging these cravings occasionally, while maintaining a nutritious diet, is important for the health of both mother and baby.

Physical discomfort, such as pain, fatigue, or stress, can also trigger food cravings. Our bodies and brains seek relief from discomfort, often through food that provides temporary distraction or comfort. Understanding this connection is vital in addressing the underlying discomfort directly, rather than resorting to unhealthy snacks.

Our circadian rhythms, which regulate our appetite and cravings, influence our food preferences throughout the day. From morning cravings for energy-boosting breakfasts to evening desires for hearty meals, our internal clocks play a significant role. Nighttime cravings, often for less healthy options, can be a product of boredom, relaxation, or hormonal changes. Structuring balanced meals and snacks throughout the day can help navigate these time-based cravings.

Habitual responses also significantly influence food cravings. Repeated associations between certain situations or emotions and specific foods can create cravings in similar future scenarios. Breaking these habits and forming healthier associations is key to overcoming such cravings.

Boredom is a notable trigger for cravings as eating provides sensory pleasure and distraction. Finding engaging activities or hobbies can be an effective strategy to prevent boredom-induced cravings. Similarly, the availability and sensory appeal of food greatly impact cravings. Creating an environment with accessible healthy options can help curb cravings for less nutritious foods.

Advertisements can also strongly influence cravings through persuasive and appealing depictions of food. Practicing media literacy and limiting exposure to such ads can help manage these induced cravings.

Lastly, drug and alcohol use, including certain medications, can trigger food cravings due to their effects on the brain and body. Understanding this connection is crucial, especially for those seeking to maintain healthy eating patterns.

Strategies for Managing Cravings

Managing food cravings effectively is a multifaceted process that requires a combination of self-awareness, cognitive strategies, dietary choices, lifestyle adjustments, and goal setting.

The cornerstone of this approach is developing craving awareness. By understanding the difference between true hunger and emotional or environmental cravings, you can make more informed choices about eating. Keeping a journal to track the specifics of your cravings, such as time and emotional state, can reveal patterns and triggers. Complementing this, mindful eating practices enable you to savor your food and recognize satiety cues, helping prevent overindulgence.

Incorporating Cognitive Behavioral Techniques (CBT) is another key strategy. CBT involves identifying and challenging negative thought patterns related to cravings. By reframing these thoughts and employing coping strategies like delaying and distracting yourself, you can resist unhealthy cravings. This approach is further supported by developing healthier mechanisms for stress management, rather than turning to food for comfort.

Focusing on satiety through dietary choices is also crucial. Consuming foods high in fiber and protein, and low in calorie density, like whole grains, fruits, vegetables, legumes, and lean proteins, can help you feel fuller and more satisfied, reducing the need for unhealthy snacking.

Hydration plays a vital role in managing cravings. Sometimes thirst is mistaken for hunger, leading to unnecessary eating. By ensuring proper hydration, you can better discern true hunger from cravings.

Meal timing is another aspect to consider. Regular, balanced meals and snacks prevent blood sugar dips that trigger cravings. Aligning meal times with daily activities, and avoiding eating close to bedtime, can also aid in craving control.

Regular exercise is a powerful tool in this process. Physical activity regulates appetite hormones, improves mood, and reduces stress, all of which help in managing cravings. Consistent exercise also builds self-discipline, enhancing overall control over eating habits.

Finally, goal setting is fundamental. Establishing specific, measurable, and realistic objectives regarding your eating habits provides clear direction. Breaking these goals into smaller steps, tracking progress, and setting non-food rewards can motivate you towards healthier choices. Remember, setbacks are part of the journey and should be used as learning opportunities.

Cravings are more than just fleeting desires; they're complex experiences influenced by physical, emotional, and environmental factors. Everything from the chemical reactions in our brains to our daily habits shapes our relationship with food.

To handle food cravings effectively, we need a holistic approach that combines mental strategies with lifestyle changes.

This approach helps us build a healthier and more balanced connection with our cravings. It's not solely about resisting temptations but also understanding why we have them and getting better at making choices that benefit both our body and overall well-being.

DINING OUT THE HEALTHY WAY

Dining out doesn't have to mean giving up on your health goals. In this section you will learn how to strike a balance between treating yourself and staying on track with your well-being. It will walk you through a variety of choices you might encounter when eating out, helping you make decisions that can either support or hinder your health objectives.

It's not just about avoiding dishes with loads of calories; it's about taking a comprehensive approach to consider nutrition, taste, and how your choices fit into your overall lifestyle. Whether you're decoding menu descriptions to uncover healthier options or picking cuisines known for their health benefits, this guide is like a map to help you navigate the diverse world of dining out.

Choosing Healthy Restaurants

Choosing healthy restaurants involves considering various factors, including the cuisine offered, the ingredients used, and the cooking methods employed. Different cuisines offer varying levels of healthiness, and understanding these can significantly enhance your dining experience.

Mediterranean cuisine is a popular healthy choice, known for its use of fruits, vegetables, whole grains, and heart-healthy fats like olive oil. It emphasizes lean proteins from fish and poultry, seasoned with a variety of herbs and spices. Japanese cuisine is another healthy option, featuring low-calorie foods rich in omega-3 fatty acids, such as sushi and sashimi. However, it's important to be mindful of high-sodium ingredients like soy sauce. Thai cuisine, with its fresh herbs, vegetables, and lean proteins, can be a flavorful and healthy choice, but watch out for high-calorie sauces and large portion sizes.

Indian cuisine offers healthy options like tandoori or grilled dishes, often including beneficial ingredients like lentils and legumes. Mexican cuisine can also be healthy if you choose dishes with grilled proteins and fresh salsa, avoiding calorie-dense items like cheese and sour cream.

Beyond specific cuisines, farm-to-table dining emphasizes fresh, locally sourced ingredients. This approach supports local farmers, reduces the carbon footprint of food transportation, and ensures meals packed with nutrients and flavor. Restaurants that focus on farm-to-table and locally sourced ingredients offer seasonal menus with a variety of fresh, nutrient-rich options.

Another key to healthy dining is carefully examining the menu. Look for items labeled as "healthy" or "light" and opt for dishes prepared using methods like grilling, baking, or steaming, which are healthier than frying. Portion sizes are also crucial; choosing smaller portions can help control calorie intake. Pay attention to the ingredients in each dish, favoring fresh, whole ingredients over those with excessive cheese or creamy sauces.

Finally, don't hesitate to ask questions at restaurants. Inquire about dietary accommodations, ingredient substitutions, portion sizes, cooking methods, and nutritional information. This will help ensure your meal aligns with your dietary needs and preferences.

Reading Restaurant Menus Wisely

Navigating restaurant menus wisely is key to making healthier dining choices. Restaurants often employ fancy jargon to describe their dishes, which can be confusing and sometimes misleading, especially when you're trying to eat healthily. Understanding these terms is crucial to avoid hidden calories and maintain a balanced diet.

Let's start with common menu terms. "Au gratin" refers to dishes baked with cheese and breadcrumbs, adding extra calories and fat. For healthier options, avoid "au gratin" dishes. "Sautéed" indicates cooking in oil or butter, which can be high in fat; ask for less oil or butter for a lighter meal. "Crusted" dishes have a coating, often made of bread, nuts, or herbs, increasing both flavor and calorie count. Consider uncrusted options if watching your intake. "Reduction" usually means a sauce simmered to concentrate flavors, potentially containing added sugar or butter. "Broiled" means cooking by direct heat and can be a healthier choice as it often uses less fat.

Hidden calories are another aspect to watch for. They sneak into meals through rich sauces, dressings, and large portion sizes. To manage this, request sauces and dressings on the side and be mindful of portion sizes, sharing meals or saving some for later. Watch out for side dishes like fries or onion rings; opt for healthier sides like steamed vegetables or salad. Also, be cautious of terms like "crispy," "fried," "battered," or "breaded," as these cooking methods significantly increase calorie content.

Balancing macronutrients is vital for a nutritious meal. Carbohydrates are essential energy sources found in foods like rice and pasta. Choose whole grains for more nutrients and fiber. Proteins are crucial for tissue repair and can be found in lean meats, tofu, and beans. Choose grilled or baked proteins over fried for less added fat. Fats are necessary but should be healthy ones found in avocados, nuts, and olive oil, avoiding dishes high in saturated and trans fats.

Choosing lean proteins is essential for muscle growth and repair. Poultry, fish, tofu, and tempeh are excellent lean protein sources. Grilled, baked, or roasted cooking methods are preferable to frying. Be aware of portion sizes to avoid overeating, even with lean proteins.

Finally, consider veggie-centric options. Salads, vegetable stir-fries, and grilled vegetable platters are nutritious choices. Opt for vinaigrettes over creamy dressings and request less oil in stir-fries. Stuffed peppers and vegetable-based pasta dishes are fulfilling options that center around vegetables.

Customizing Your Order

Dining out while trying to make healthier choices can be challenging, but understanding how to customize your order can make a significant difference. Special dietary requests and substitutions are key strategies to ensure your meal aligns with your health goals, whether you're dealing with food allergies, dietary restrictions, or simply aiming for a healthier lifestyle.

Communicating your needs clearly to restaurant staff is crucial, especially for specific health conditions like celiac disease, lactose intolerance, or food allergies. Requests for gluten-free, dairy-free, vegetarian, or vegan options are increasingly common and most restaurants are equipped to accommodate them. For instance, gluten-free pasta or dairy-free cheese alternatives can be requested to cater to specific dietary needs.

Substitutions are another effective way to tailor your meal. Swapping high-calorie sides for healthier options, such as replacing french fries with a side salad, can significantly reduce calorie intake. Similarly, opting for lettuce wraps instead of bread or zucchini noodles in place of traditional pasta can benefit those on low-carb or gluten-free diets. Requesting grilled or baked dishes over fried ones can also cut down on unhealthy fats and calories.

Another simple yet effective strategy is to request sauces and dressings on the side. This control over condiments helps manage calorie and fat intake. For salads, a light toss of dressing or a drizzle on the side can make a big difference, while for main courses, the option to add sauces sparingly allows for a healthier meal without sacrificing taste.

Customized salads offer a fantastic opportunity to control the nutritional content of your meal. Starting with a base of fresh greens and adding toppings like vegetables, fruits, nuts, and lean proteins can create a nutritious and satisfying meal. Being mindful of portion sizes and choosing lighter dressings can further enhance the health benefits of a customized salad.

Paying attention to sugar and sodium content is also important. Requesting dishes with less or no added sugar, and opting for low-sodium options, helps in maintaining a balanced diet. Choosing naturally low-sugar and low-sodium dishes, like grilled meats and fresh fruits, can also contribute to a healthier dining experience.

You now know how to spot the healthier options in a wide range of foods and have a bunch of strategies to use. From picking cuisines that align with your health goals to customizing your orders to match your dietary needs. Remember, eating out healthily isn't just a one-time decision; it's a rewarding way of life. Use these tips and insights as you keep discovering new foods, making sure each meal satisfies your taste buds while also nourishing your body.

HEALTHY EATING FOR SPECIAL DIETS

In this section, you will learn how to apply the fundamental principles of nutrition to make choices that align with dietary restrictions, such as gluten-free, dairy-free, or a plant-based diet. It not only provides information on what to eat but also offers practical advice on how to make informed and healthy choices.

Food Allergies and Intolerances

Understanding the differences between food allergies and intolerances is crucial for managing our diets and health effectively. Food allergies involve the immune system reacting strongly to certain foods, mistakenly identifying harmless proteins as threats. This can lead to symptoms like hives, swelling, and in severe cases, anaphylaxis, which are typically rapid and potentially life-threatening.

Conversely, food intolerances, such as lactose intolerance, arise from the digestive system's inability to process certain foods, leading to symptoms like bloating and diarrhea. These reactions are generally less severe and not life-threatening.

Key distinctions between the two include the reaction time and severity. Allergies usually prompt immediate reactions, while intolerances can have delayed symptoms. Allergies can be severe and life-threatening, whereas intolerances mainly cause discomfort.

For those with allergies, avoidance of trigger foods and carrying an epinephrine auto-injector is vital. People with intolerances may tolerate small amounts of the problem food or find relief with enzyme supplements.

Several foods are more likely to cause allergies, including peanuts, tree nuts, milk, eggs, wheat, soy, fish, shellfish, and sesame. Awareness of these common allergens is essential for preventing allergic reactions.

Recognizing allergic reactions is also crucial. Symptoms can range from skin issues like hives to respiratory problems, digestive discomfort, and in severe cases, anaphylaxis. Timely medical intervention and use of prescribed epinephrine auto-injectors are important for managing these reactions.

Diagnosing these conditions involves medical history review, physical examinations, and tests like skin prick tests, blood tests, and oral food challenges for allergies. For intolerances, tests like lactose tolerance and breath tests, or elimination diets, are common.

For individuals with these conditions, reading food labels is essential. This involves checking ingredient lists, allergen statements, cross-contamination warnings, and understanding terms like "gluten-free." Nutritional content and serving sizes are also key for those with specific dietary needs.

When cooking for those with allergies or intolerances, ingredient substitution is key. Using alternatives like gluten-free flours or plant-based milks and ensuring a clean cooking environment to prevent cross-contamination is crucial. Communication of dietary needs when dining out or attending social gatherings is also important.

For those dining out or traveling, planning is key. This includes communicating dietary restrictions to restaurants, choosing establishments that specialize in allergy-friendly cuisine, and carrying necessary medications. Researching dining options, packing safe snacks, and cooking your meals when possible can also help manage these conditions while traveling.

Gluten-Free Eating

Gluten-free diets have surged in popularity, extending beyond those with celiac disease to include individuals with gluten intolerance and sensitivity. This uptick in gluten-free eating is attributed to a heightened awareness of gluten-related discomforts and the influence of social media, which offers abundant resources, recipes, and personal experiences regarding gluten-free lifestyles. The food industry has responded by broadening the range of gluten-free products, making it easier for individuals to adopt such diets. Additionally, many people perceive gluten-free diets as healthier, associating them with benefits like weight loss or improved well-being, even in the absence of medical justifications.

While gluten-free diets are essential for those with celiac disease or gluten sensitivity, it's important to recognize that they may not offer additional health benefits for everyone. In fact, some gluten-free products could be less nutritious due to alternative flours and additives used to replicate the taste and texture of traditional foods. Thus, it's critical for individuals to make informed dietary decisions and consult healthcare professionals if they suspect gluten intolerance or sensitivity.

One must be aware of hidden gluten sources to effectively maintain a gluten-free diet. Gluten can unexpectedly appear in sauces, condiments, processed foods, and beverages. For example, soy sauce often contains wheat, and many processed foods use wheat flour as a thickener. Cross-contamination is also a concern, whether in shared kitchen spaces, restaurants, or through utensils and cutting boards. Alcoholic beverages like beer, as well as some flavored coffees and teas, might also contain gluten. Carefully reading labels and asking questions when dining out are key practices for those adhering to a gluten-free diet.

The benefits of a gluten-free diet primarily apply to individuals with celiac disease or gluten sensitivity. These people may experience improved well-being and digestive health upon eliminating gluten. Some also report increased energy and better digestion, often because a gluten-free diet can lead to consuming fewer processed foods. However, potential downsides include nutrient deficiencies, particularly if gluten-containing grains are not properly substituted with nutritious alternatives. Over-reliance on processed gluten-free products can lead to unhealthy dietary habits, and dining out can present challenges due to cross-contamination risks.

To maintain nutritional balance, it's essential to find nutritious alternatives to traditional grains. Options like brown rice, quinoa, buckwheat, amaranth, and millet offer a range of nutrients and can be incorporated into a diverse diet. Remember to choose certified gluten-free grains to avoid cross-contamination. Additionally, attention should be paid to fiber, iron, calcium, and vitamin B12 intake to avoid deficiencies common in gluten-free diets. This can be achieved through a balanced diet that includes fruits, vegetables, lean proteins, and fortified products.

Dairy-Free and Lactose-Free Diets

Lactose intolerance, a condition affecting many worldwide, involves difficulty in digesting lactose, a natural sugar found in dairy products like milk, cheese, and yogurt. The key enzyme, lactase, is essential for breaking down lactose into simpler sugars for absorption. However, those lacking adequate lactase experience symptoms like bloating, gas, diarrhea, and stomach cramps upon consuming dairy. This intolerance varies; some tolerate small lactose amounts, while others must avoid it entirely. It often stems from genetic predisposition or secondary causes like celiac disease or Crohn's disease. Diagnosis and management guidance from healthcare professionals are crucial.

Managing lactose intolerance involves dietary modifications, including reducing dairy intake and opting for lactose-free or dairy-free alternatives like almond milk, soy milk, and lactose-free yogurt. It's crucial to distinguish between lactose-free and dairy-free diets. The former avoids lactose for those with intolerance, while the latter excludes all dairy products, often due to allergies or ethical reasons.

Additionally, those on these diets must be cautious of hidden lactose sources in processed foods, medications, and certain restaurant dishes. Vigilant label reading and inquiring about ingredients are key to avoiding such hidden lactose.

Nutritional considerations are vital, as dairy-free and lactose-free diets can lead to deficiencies in calcium, vitamin D, protein, and vitamin B12. Fortified non-dairy alternatives and dietary diversity can help mitigate these risks. Consulting healthcare professionals ensures balanced nutrition while adhering to these diets.

Cooking without dairy offers a chance to explore a variety of dairy-free substitutes and flavors. Non-dairy milks, dairy-free margarine, and cheese alternatives can replace traditional dairy products in cooking and baking. Emphasizing herbs, spices, and plant-based seasonings can enhance flavor and nutritional value.

Plant-Based and Vegetarian Diets

The discussion of plant-based and vegetarian diets encompasses a range of dietary choices centered on plant foods like vegetables, fruits, grains, nuts, seeds, and legumes. Plant-based diets primarily focus on these foods while minimizing or completely avoiding animal products, such as meat, dairy, and eggs. Individuals choose this diet for health, environmental, and ethical reasons, and it offers flexibility to adjust animal product intake according to personal preferences and health goals.

Conversely, vegetarian diets are more specific. They exclude meat, poultry, and seafood but include other animal-derived foods like dairy and eggs. Some vegetarians might choose to include or exclude certain animal byproducts based on their personal beliefs. Both diets emphasize plant foods and reduce meat consumption, offering health benefits like lower risks of heart disease, diabetes, and certain cancers, and have a smaller environmental footprint.

Plant-based diets offer numerous health benefits, including a reduced risk of chronic diseases, better weight management, diabetes management and prevention, potential cancer-fighting properties, and improved digestive health. These diets are rich in vitamins, minerals, fiber, and antioxidants, enhancing overall health and well-being.

For vegetarians, careful planning is necessary to meet dietary needs. Protein is essential and various plant-based foods fulfill this need.

Legumes, nuts, seeds, tofu, tempeh, whole grains, leafy greens, and plant-based protein powders are excellent protein sources. Iron absorption can be enhanced by pairing iron-rich foods with vitamin C-rich foods, such as lentils for iron with bell peppers for vitamin C. Calcium sources include fortified plant-based milk, leafy greens, almonds, and tofu. Vitamin B12 can be obtained from fortified foods and supplements, and omega-3 fatty acids from flaxseeds, chia seeds, walnuts, and hemp seeds.

Transitioning to a plant-based diet is a significant dietary shift that often requires a gradual adjustment to ensure both nutritional adequacy and long-term sustainability. This process involves reducing the consumption of animal products while incorporating a wider variety of plant-based foods into your daily meals. It's important to recognize that this journey can be a learning experience, and understanding your nutritional needs is essential to make informed dietary choices.

One of the key aspects of transitioning to a plant-based diet is meal planning. This involves not only identifying sources of plant-based protein but also ensuring a balanced intake of vitamins, minerals, and other essential nutrients. By planning meals and snacks ahead of time, you can create well-rounded and satisfying plant-based meals that meet your dietary requirements.

Plant-based alternatives play a significant role in easing the transition. There are now a plethora of plant-based substitutes available for traditional animal products, such as plant-based milk, tofu, tempeh, and meat alternatives. These substitutes can be used in familiar recipes to recreate the flavors and textures that you may be accustomed to from animal-based foods.

Seeking support from the plant-based community or like-minded individuals can be beneficial during the transition. Online forums, social media groups, and local vegetarian or vegan organizations provide opportunities to connect with others who have similar dietary goals. Sharing experiences, recipes, and advice with a supportive community can make the transition more enjoyable and less daunting.

Finally, remember that patience is a virtue. It's common to encounter challenges along the way, whether they relate to adjusting to new flavors and textures or navigating social situations where animal products are prevalent. Recognizing that dietary changes take time and that it's okay to make mistakes along the way can help alleviate stress and frustration.

Diabetes-Friendly Eating

Diabetes is a widespread health condition that affects how your body uses glucose, a vital energy source derived from the food we consume. Our digestive system breaks down the carbohydrates in food into glucose, which enters our bloodstream. Insulin, a hormone produced by the pancreas, facilitates the entry of glucose into our cells for energy. However, diabetes disrupts this process.

There are two main types of diabetes. Type 1 and Type 2. Type 1 diabetes occurs when the body's immune system attacks the insulin-producing cells in the pancreas, leading to a lack of insulin and high blood sugar levels. People with Type 1 diabetes need to take insulin externally. Type 2 diabetes, which is more common, arises when the body's cells resist insulin's effects or when the pancreas struggles to produce enough insulin, also leading to high blood sugar levels.

Unmanaged high blood sugar can lead to severe health issues like heart disease, kidney disease, vision problems, and nerve damage. Therefore, managing diabetes effectively is crucial for those affected.

A key aspect of diabetes management is maintaining blood sugar levels within a healthy range, primarily through diet. Paying attention to carbohydrate intake is vital, as carbohydrates convert into glucose in the bloodstream. Spreading carbohydrate consumption evenly throughout the day helps avoid blood sugar spikes. Including fiber-rich foods like whole grains, vegetables, and legumes is beneficial, as fiber slows carbohydrate absorption, stabilizing blood sugar levels. Protein intake from sources like lean meats, poultry, fish, tofu, and beans can also help control blood sugar.

Portion control is essential; overeating can cause blood sugar spikes, even with healthy foods. Regular monitoring of blood sugar levels, with guidance from healthcare providers, helps individuals understand how different foods affect their blood sugar.

Carbohydrate counting is another effective tool for managing blood sugar. It involves tracking the carbohydrates in meals and snacks, as they significantly impact blood sugar. This approach offers meal planning flexibility and helps adjust insulin or medication doses based on carbohydrate intake. Learning about portion sizes and carbohydrate content in foods is necessary for accurate tracking.

The glycemic index (GI) is a helpful tool in selecting appropriate foods. It ranks foods based on their effect on blood sugar levels. Low GI foods (score of 55 or less) cause gradual blood sugar increases, while high GI foods (score above 70) lead to rapid spikes. Moderate GI foods fall in between. Incorporating low and moderate GI foods and limiting high GI foods is beneficial for blood sugar control.

Fiber is particularly important in a diabetes-friendly diet. It slows carbohydrate digestion and absorption, preventing rapid blood sugar spikes. Soluble fiber, found in foods like oats, barley, beans, and certain fruits, improves insulin sensitivity. Insoluble fiber aids digestive health and is found in foods like whole grains and vegetables. A high-fiber diet also supports weight management and reduces heart disease risk, both important for people with diabetes.

Heart-Healthy Eating

Maintaining a healthy heart is critical for overall well-being, and a heart-healthy diet plays a pivotal role in achieving this. A balanced diet that includes specific nutrients is key to promoting heart health.

Fiber, particularly soluble fiber found in whole grains, fruits, vegetables, and legumes, is essential for lowering "bad" cholesterol (LDL) levels and controlling blood sugar. Omega-3 fatty acids, present in fatty fish like salmon, mackerel, trout, flaxseeds, and walnuts, offer anti-inflammatory benefits and help reduce heart disease risks by lowering blood pressure and preventing arterial plaque buildup.

Antioxidants, including vitamins C and E, protect blood vessels from free radical damage and reduce inflammation. Sources of these antioxidants are citrus fruits, strawberries, nuts, and seeds. Potassium, a mineral in bananas, oranges, spinach, and potatoes, helps regulate blood pressure and reduces heart strain.

Reducing sodium intake is also crucial for heart health. Excess sodium can lead to high blood pressure, a significant heart disease risk factor. Limiting salt in cooking and choosing "low-sodium" or "sodium-free" products helps manage sodium levels. When dining out, opting for dishes with less salt and avoiding high-sodium processed and packaged foods are beneficial practices.

The Mediterranean Diet, inspired by traditional eating habits around the Mediterranean Sea, is recognized for its heart-healthy benefits. It emphasizes fresh fruits and vegetables, olive oil as a primary fat source, whole grains, lean proteins like fish and seafood, and nuts and seeds. This diet minimizes processed and sugary foods, promoting overall heart health.

The DASH Diet, designed to lower high blood pressure, focuses on reducing sodium intake and consuming potassium, calcium, and magnesium-rich foods. It encourages eating fruits, vegetables, whole grains, lean proteins, and healthy fats while limiting saturated and trans fats.

Managing cholesterol levels is another critical component of maintaining heart health. The goal is to lower levels of "bad" cholesterol, known as low-density lipoprotein (LDL), while increasing levels of "good" cholesterol, called high-density lipoprotein (HDL).

To reduce LDL cholesterol, minimize the intake of saturated and trans fats in your diet. Saturated fats are commonly found in animal products like red meat, butter, and full-fat dairy products, as well as in some tropical oils like coconut and palm oil. Trans fats are often found in partially hydrogenated oils, which are used in many processed and fried foods.

Conversely, including heart-healthy fats in your diet is essential for promoting cardiovascular health. Monounsaturated and polyunsaturated fats, found in foods like olive oil, avocados, nuts, and seeds, can help raise HDL cholesterol and lower LDL cholesterol when they replace saturated and trans fats. Omega-3 fatty acids, which are abundant in fatty fish like salmon, mackerel, and trout, also have a positive effect on cholesterol levels and overall heart health.

Soluble fiber is another dietary component that can contribute to cholesterol management. Foods rich in soluble fiber, such as oats, barley, beans, lentils, fruits, and vegetables, can help reduce LDL cholesterol levels by binding to cholesterol in the digestive tract and facilitating its removal from the body.

Plant sterols and stanols, naturally present in select plant-based foods like soybeans, broccoli, and almonds, as well as fortified products, play a pivotal role in the management of cholesterol levels. These compounds bear a resemblance to cholesterol in their chemical structure and offer the potential to impede the absorption of cholesterol in the intestines. When integrated into a well-rounded diet, they contribute to the reduction of LDL cholesterol levels.

Heart-healthy cooking techniques also play a crucial role. Steaming, grilling, baking, stir-frying, and poaching are excellent methods that preserve nutrients and reduce unhealthy fats and calories. Using herbs, spices, and citrus fruits enhances flavors without adding unhealthy ingredients.

CONSEQUENCES OF A POOR DIET

As you have learned, a balanced diet, rich in essential nutrients, is the cornerstone of good health. Conversely, poor dietary habits can lead to myriad health issues. A whole book could be written about the consequences of a poor diet. Instead, this chapter provides an overview of some common ways a poor diet can negatively impact your health. Consider this chapter a reminder of why it's important to adopt the healthy eating behaviors presented so far.

Our energy levels are greatly influenced by the quality of our diet. When we consume too many sugary or processed foods, it can lead to a quick energy boost followed by a crash, leaving us feeling tired. Nutrient deficiencies, like not getting enough iron, can cause a condition called anemia, which is characterized by weakness and exhaustion. Insufficient intake of vitamins such as B12 and D can also have a negative impact on our energy and overall well-being.

Furthermore, our diet can affect the health of our bones. If we don't get enough vitamin D, we increase our risk of osteoporosis, and a lack of calcium can also result in weaker bones. On the flip side, excessive consumption of sodium, caffeine, and alcohol can harm our bone health.

Our dietary choices also play a significant role in our digestive health. Not eating enough fiber, which is often the case with poor diets, can lead to issues like constipation, bloating, and discomfort. Overindulging in processed and fatty foods can raise the risk of heartburn and acid reflux. These eating habits can also trigger gastrointestinal disorders such as irritable bowel syndrome (IBS) and contribute to inflammation in the digestive tract.

Our skin's health is closely tied to our diet as well. A less-than-ideal diet can lead to skin problems like acne, dryness, and premature aging. Essential nutrients like vitamins A, C, and E, along with Omega-3 fatty acids, are crucial for maintaining skin elasticity and hydration.

The link between our diet and mental health is also substantial. Diets high in sugar and processed foods can result in mood swings and an increased risk of depression and anxiety. A healthy gut microbiome, influenced by our diet, is essential for our mental well-being. Nutrient-rich diets that include Omega-3 fatty acids and B vitamins support mood regulation and cognitive function.

Our dietary habits significantly impact the risk of hypertension or high blood pressure, which is often associated with excessive salt intake. Reducing salt and adopting a balanced diet can help manage blood pressure.

Unhealthy dietary choices raise the risk of cardiovascular diseases such as heart disease and stroke. Foods that are high in unhealthy fats can raise LDL cholesterol, while excessive salt intake contributes to high blood pressure. A heart-healthy diet that is rich in fiber, antioxidants, and omega-3 fatty acids can help prevent these diseases.

Diets that are high in sugar and refined carbohydrates increase the risk of Type 2 diabetes by causing insulin resistance. Obesity, often resulting from poor diet, further increases this risk. A balanced diet can help stabilize blood sugar levels and reduce the risk of diabetes.

Obesity, which occurs when we consume more calories than we burn, poses health risks for both adults and children. It increases the likelihood of developing conditions such as Type 2 diabetes, heart disease, and joint problems. In children, obesity can lead to social and emotional challenges, as well as long-term health issues. Preventing obesity involves adopting healthier eating habits and increasing physical activity.

The significant role of diet in shaping our overall health cannot be overstated. The choices we make at the dining table extend far beyond mere satisfaction of hunger; they play a critical role in determining our energy levels, skin health, bone strength, and even our mental state.

Poor dietary habits can set the stage for chronic diseases, including heart disease, diabetes, and obesity, while a balanced and nutritious diet can be a powerful tool in preventing these conditions. Embracing a diet rich in essential nutrients is not just a step towards better health, but a journey towards a more fulfilling and vibrant life.

CONCLUSION

The path to developing and maintaining healthy eating behaviors is not a one-time effort, but rather a continuous process of learning and adaptation. This guide has provided you with foundational knowledge in nutrition, tools for making informed choices, and strategies to navigate the complexities of eating well in various aspects of life.

From understanding the fundamentals of nutrition to recognizing the pitfalls of fad diets, this journey has been about equipping you with the knowledge to make healthier choices. The art of effective grocery shopping and the skills for meal planning and preparation are not just techniques; they are empowering tools that enable you to take control of your diet and health.

We've also tackled the emotional aspects of eating, acknowledging that food cravings and emotional eating are common experiences. By understanding these triggers and learning strategies to manage them, you are better positioned to maintain your nutrition goals, even when faced with challenges.

Remember, dining out and enjoying social meals are part of a fulfilling life. This guide has shown you that these can be harmonious with your health goals. For those on special diets, the journey is the same, with some additional considerations to ensure your needs are met.

As you move forward, keep in mind that each section of this guide is not just a standalone piece of information, but a part of a comprehensive approach to a healthier lifestyle. The knowledge you've gained here is a solid foundation, and the steps you take next are crucial for continuing the journey towards a healthier, happier life.

THANKS FOR READING

Dear reader,

Thank you for reading *Eat Smart for Life: A Guide to Developing Healthy Eating Behaviors.*

If you enjoyed this book, please leave a review where you bought it. It helps more than most people think.

Get the Healthy Eating Bundle For FREE!

www.FunctionalHealth.Coach/Healthy-Eating-Bundle-Free

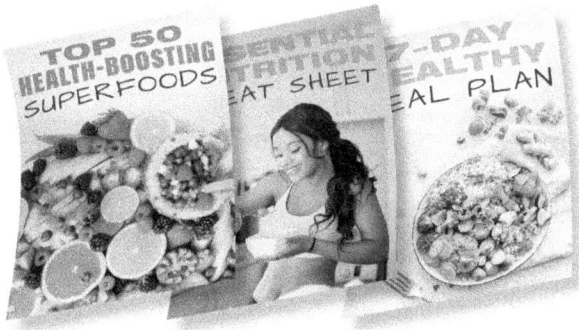

Includes:

- Top 50 Health-Boosting Superfoods
- Essential Nutrition Cheat Sheet
- 7-Day Healthy Meal Plan

Get them all FREE here: www.FunctionalHealth.-Coach/Healthy-Eating-Bundle-Free

ABOUT SAM FURY

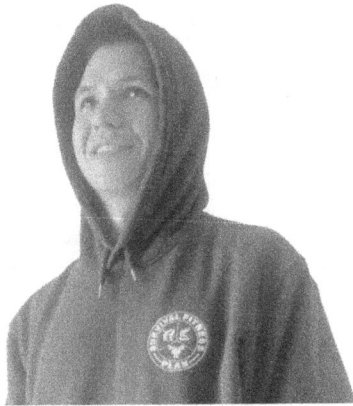

Health Coach - Content Creator - Optimist

www.SamFury.com

amazon.com/author/samfury

goodreads.com/SamFury

facebook.com/SamFuryOfficial

instagram.com/samfuryofficial

youtube.com/@FunctionalHealthShow

REFERENCES

https://aaaai.org

https://aafa.org

https://acog.org

https://agreenerworld.org

https://allergicliving.com

https://allrecipes.com

https://amazon.com

https://americanpregnancy.org

https://ams.usda.gov

https://apa.org

https://apps.who.int

https://archive.org

https://asc-aqua.org

https://cambridge.org

https://catalog.oslri.net

https://cdc.gov

https://certifiedhumane.org

https://choosemyplate.gov

https://ciwf.org

https://clark.com

https://consumerreports.org

https://cookinglight.com

https://diabetes.org

https://dietaryguidelines.gov

https://doi.org

https://earthday.org

https://eatright.org

https://eatrightontario.ca

https://epa.gov

https://ethicalconsumer.org

https://fairtradecertified.org

http://fao.org

https://fda.gov

https://feedingamerica.org

https://foodallergy.org

https://foodethicscouncil.org

https://foodnetwork.com

https://foodtank.com

https://forbes.com

https://fruitsandveggiesmorematters.org

https://fsis.usda.gov

https://greatist.com

https://health.harvard.edu

https://healthlibrary.uhc.com

https://healthline.com

https://heart.org

https://hindawi.com

https://hsph.harvard.edu

https://iatp.org

https://iffgd.org

https://ift.org

https://kidswithfoodallergies.org

https://liberalarts.uoregon.edu

https://lipidworld.biomedcentral.com

https://lovefoodhatewaste.com

https://lpi.oregonstate.edu

https://mayoclinic.org

https://mayoclinic.org

https://medicalnewstoday.com

https://medlineplus.gov

https://msc.org

https://msc.org

https://myplate.gov

https://nationalgeographic.com

https://nature.com

https://nhlbi.nih.gov

https://nia.nih.gov

https://niaid.nih.gov

https://niams.nih.gov

https://niddk.nih.gov

https://nimh.nih.gov

https://nof.org

https://nongmoproject.org

https://ods.od.nih.gov

https://ota.com

https://perlego.com

https://psycnet.apa.org

https://pubmed.ncbi.nlm.nih.gov

https://rainforest-alliance.org

https://researchgate.net/publication

https://scirp.org

https://sdgs.un.org

https://seafoodwatch.org

https://search.worldcat.org

https://sustainablefoodtrust.org

https://sutterhealth.org

https://thegoodtrade.com

https://theguardian.com

https://us.fsc.org

https://verywellfit.com

https://vrg.org

https://washington.edu

https://wcrf.org

https://webmd.com

https://who.int/news-room/fact-sheets/detail/obesity-and-over
weight

https://world-heart-federation.org